KETO DINNER

Discover 30 Easy to Follow Ketogenic Cookbook Dinner recipes for Your Low-Carb Diet with Gluten-Free and wheat to Maximize your weight loss

STEPHANIE BAKER

CURRIED COCONUT WITH SPINACH LEAVES

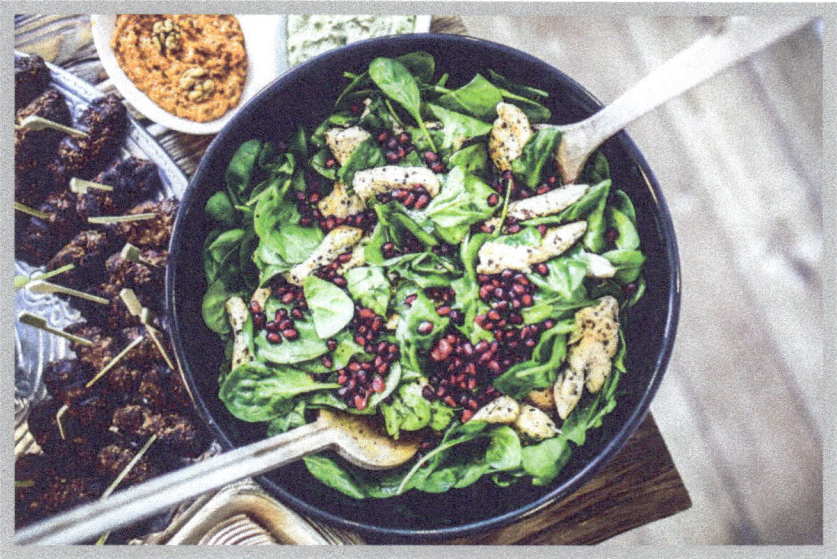

30 MINUTES

Serving 2

INGREDIENTS

- 450 g Leaves of Frozen Spinach
- 380 grams of coconut milk
- Curry pulp 1-2 tsp yellow (or 1-2 tsp curry powder)
- ½ Salted Teaspoon
- 1 Skin Lemon Teaspoon
- Optional: grain pomegranates
- Optional: fillet, fried chicken

PREPARATION

1. Prepare the spinach according to directions on the box.
2. Get a middle scale pan and then let it heat up a little. Add 2 yellow curry paste teaspoons and a few coconut milk spoons to the pan and stir well until a homogeneous sauce is formed.
3. Let it simmer for a couple minutes.
4. Add the prepared spinach and coconut milk remaining. It all mix well together.
5. Let it all cook before the sauce gets thick.
6. Garnish the ketogenic platter with almonds, cashews or dry fruit if you like.

LASANGE ZUCCHINI

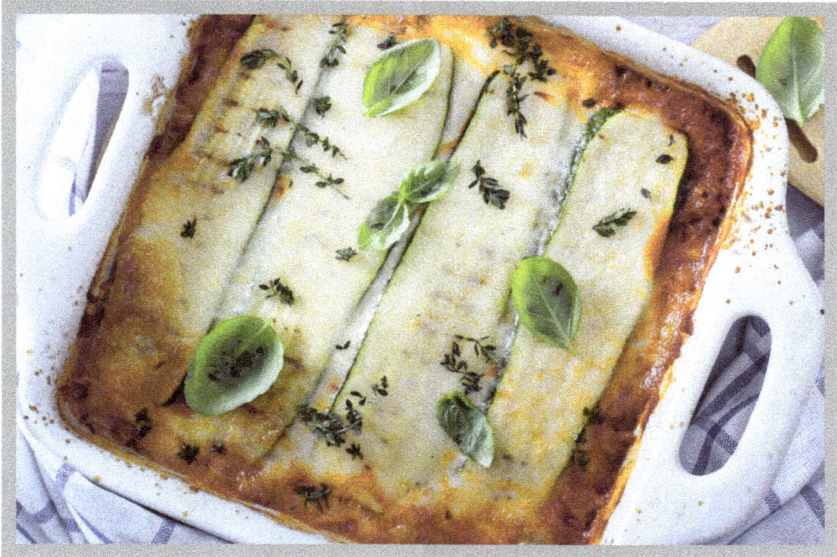

30 MINUTES

Serving 4

INGREDIENTS

- 450 g slightly lean beef
- 1 1/2 salt
- 1 Tinpoon of olive oil
- 1/2 Onion, thinly sliced
- 1 Clove of finely chopped garlic
- Tomatoes 1 may, Chunky
- 2 tbsp fresh, finely chopped basil
- Black Chickpeas
- 3 Medium size courgettes-cut into medium-thin longitudinal slices
- 1 1/2 cups of cheese with ricotta
- Parmesan cheese: 1/4 cup, rubbed
- 1 Egg (figure L)
- 400 g Mozzarella, rubberized

PREPARATION

1. Fry the onion and garlic in the olive oil pan for 2 minutes. Remove the carnivores. Once the meat isn't pink anymore, add the tomato can, basil, salt and pepper.
2. Let all cool down for about 30-40 minutes at low heat. Dilute the sauce with a little water, if the sauce is too thick.
3. Meanwhile, cut the courgettes into 1/8 thick slices (lengthways) and slightly salt both sides (the salt will drain the courgettes a bit).
4. Dab the zucchini slices off a kitchen roll with a bit of paper after 10 minutes.
5. Fry the slices of zucchini lightly on each side, really only very briefly, until they have browned slightly.

6. Insert the slices onto paper towels to remove the excess liquid.

7. Oven preheat to 190 ° C.

8. Mix the ricotta cheese, parmesan and egg in a medium saucepan.

9. Consider taking a baking dish of 9 x 12, and line the bottom with slices of zucchini. Spread the zucchini over ketogenic tomato and meat sauce.

10. Attach half a cup of the ricotta mixture and cheese to sauce. Sprinkle 1 cup of the cheese with mozzarella on top. Layer it all together before supplies run dry.

11. Before the mozzarella the last layer will go into the oven first. Cover aluminum foil to the baking dish.

12. Sprinkle 1 cup of the mozzarella onto the lasagne after 20 minutes. Bake it all 10 minutes over again.

13. Let the dinner cool down a bit before serving the ketogenic lasagna.

3

CHEESEBURGERS WITH BACON AND CHEESE FILLING

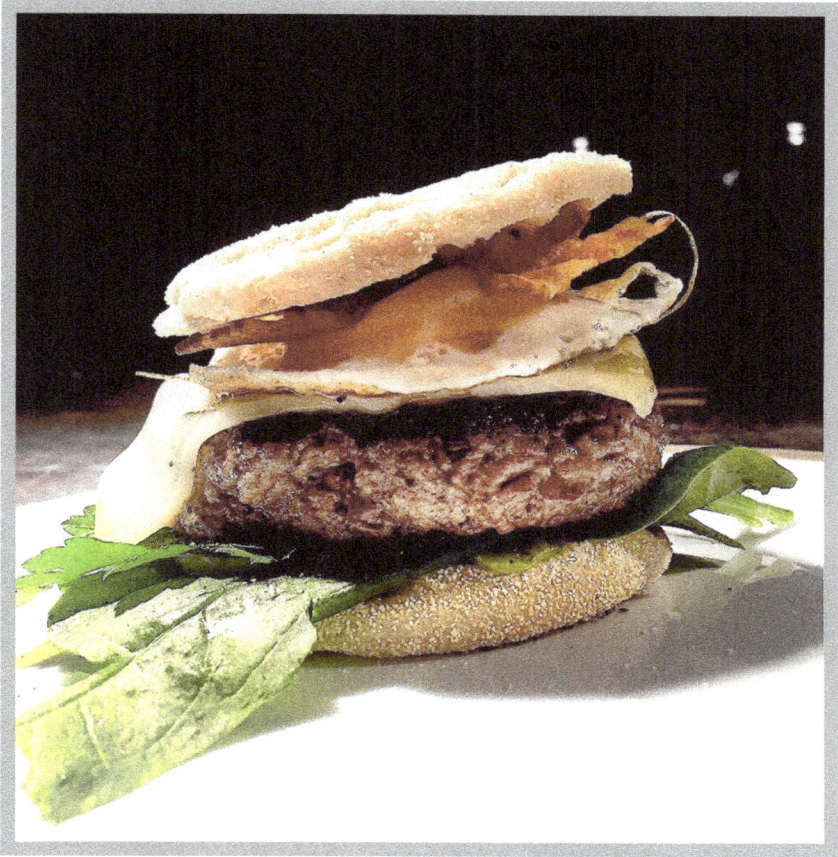

30 MINUTES

Serving 2

INGREDIENTS

- 230 g Boiled Beef
- 2 Bacon Slices

- Mozzarella: 30 g
- 55 g, sliced cheddar

- 1 Tablespoon of salt

- 1/2 Teaspoon chili pepper

- 1 Cajun teaspoon powder

- 1 cup of butter, or ghee

- Wolfbrot

- Cloud Bread Ingredients:

- 2 Eggs 2 Eggs

- 3 Tbsp of cream cheese (goat tastes really good:-)

- Baking Powder 1/4 tsp

PREPARATION

1. Cloud Bread Preparedness

1. Beat the egg whites to hard, first.

1. Mix egg yolk and baking powder into the cream cheese.

1. Fold in the whites of the egg and lightly mix again.

1. You can either sweet or salty the ketogenic cloud bread by either seasoning it with salt & pepper or sweetening it with stevia liquid, then it becomes more of a brioche.

1. Form portions of the same size and bake the ketogenic rolls about 20-30 minutes at 150 ° C. Ultimately, put some baking paper over it so it isn't getting too dark on top.

1. Blend well the minced meat and all the spices.

1. Structure patties of the meat that has been minced.

1. Load the meat with mozzarella so as not to see the cheese.

1. In a saucepan, put 1 tbsp butter or ghee and heat.

1. Put the patties in the saucepan. Fry meat for approximately 3 minutes. Flip the ketogenic patties and now top with the cheddar cheese.

1. Fry another 2-3 minutes on the meat. Take off pan the finished burgers.

1. Bacon fry.

1. Put the fried bacon onto the ketogenic burger diet.

(4)

PESTO SHRIMP GRILLED ON A STICK

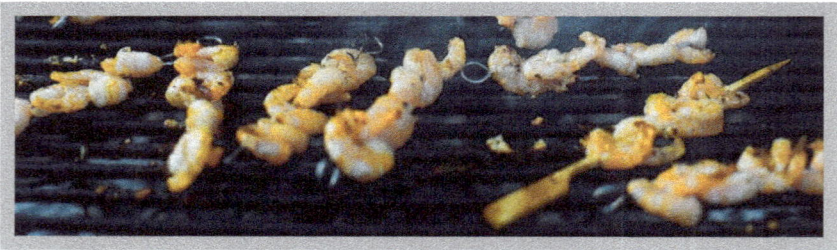

2O MINUTES

Serving 2

INGREDIENTS

- 1/2 cup basil
- 1 A small garlic clove
- 1 Tbsp of roasted pine nuts
- 2 Tbsp Parmesan, rubbed
- Olive oil: 2 tbsp

- 1 Tbsp lemon juice-preferably the new lemon juice
- Season with salt and pepper
- 450 g shrimps-ready for feeding

PREPARATION

1. In a blender, placed the basil, garlic, roasted pine nuts, parmesan, butter, lemon juice , salt and pepper until a fine pesto is obtained.
2. Marinate the shrimp now with the pesto and put the marinated shrimps in the refrigerator for at least 20 minutes.
3. Skewer the prawns on wooden sticks, fry or grill the skewers in a saucepan or grill over medium heat (about 2-3 minutes per side).

CHAMPIGNON EGGPLANT AND BACON ALLA ALFREDO

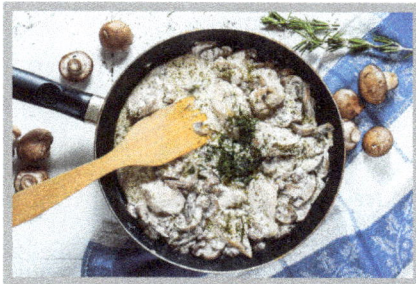

15 minutes

Serving 4

INGREDIENTS

- Bacon: 450 g
- 380 g Aubergine
- 300 g Champions gray
- 1 Cup of crème
- 2 Cups of butter
- 2 Ail cloves, rubbed in
- 1 cup of white wine
- 1 cup of lemon juice
- 1 Cup of grated Parmesan cheese
- New basil

PREPARATION

1. Cut the bacon and fry over medium heat in a large saucepan.
2. Remove the bacon from the pan as soon as it becomes crispy, and place it on kitchen paper to absorb the liquid.
3. Extract the eggplant, cut the bacon fat into strips, and heat until it becomes soft.
4. Consider making a kule in the middle of the pan-thus push the edge of the aubergine strips-and add 2 butter spoons.
5. Once the butter has melted, add the garlic and stir all together.
6. Stir in the cream, white wine and a fresh lemon juice and mix.
7. Sprinkle the rubbed parmesan over the eggplant-cream mixture and mix again.
8. Put 1/2 of the fried bacon to the saucepan and allow to simmer for 2-5 minutes.

9. The dish is then garnished with the bacon and fresh basil left over.

TUNA STEAK WITH RED BELL PEPPER AND AVOCADO SALSA

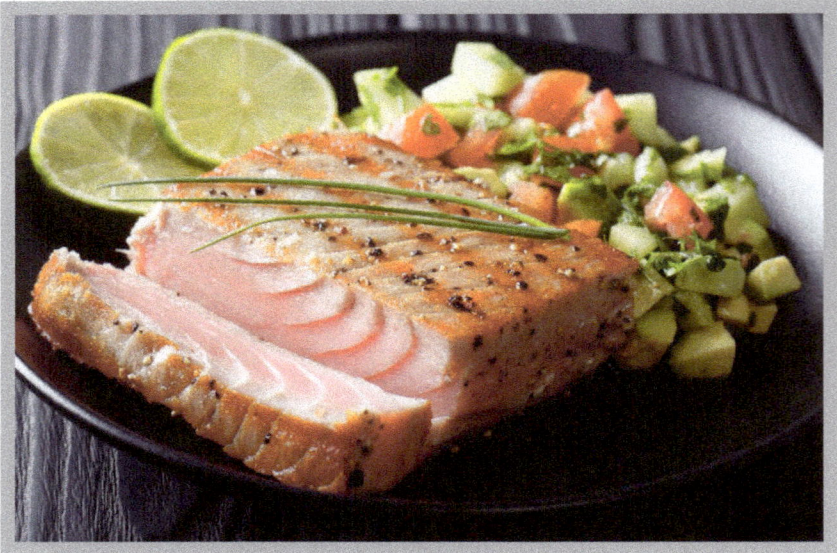

45 MINUTES

Serving 2

INGREDIENTS

- 4 Tbsp ghee or coconut oil
- 1 Half red onion
- 1 Medium Red Potato
- 2/3 cups of sweet paprika, powder
- Cumin 2/3 teaspoon, Powder
- A tablespoon of pepper flakes
- 1 A garlic clove
- 1 Tbsp cider apple vinegar

The Steak Tuna Ingredients:

- 1 Tbsp coconut oil or macadamia oil
- A little Olive Oil
- 1 cup of butter, or ghee
- 1 Spoonful of coriander seeds
- 2 Tuna steaks (150 g each)
- 1 Lime Tail
- Pinch salt and chili pepper
- Ingredients for Salsa Avocado:
- 1 Great Mature Avocado
- 2 Tbsp fresh, chopped coriander
- A little new lime juice
- A splash of water

PREPARATION

1. Clean the steaks from the tuna, dry them well, season with salt and pepper and drizzle on both sides with olive oil.
2. Put aside so room temperature comes in.
3. Heat 4 spoonfuls of coconut oil in a saucepan and add

onions and red peppers.

4. Cover with a lock, and cook for five minutes.
5. Now add to the pan the paprika powder, cumin, garlic, salt, chilli flakes, apple cider vinegar and 2 table spoons of water.
6. Mix all together and cook for another 5-7 minutes, until all is soft and nice.
7. Pour the tuna steaks into a tub so that the pans can be used.
8. Use a mortar to crush coriander seeds, or use coriander powder.
9. Warm the pan with macadamia or coconut oil, and butter or ghee.
10. Then add the coriander and the lime zest.
11. Position the steaks of the tuna into the pan and cook both sides over medium heat. Sprinkle with the lime juice over the tuna steaks in between While the avocado salsa can be prepared.
12. Cut the skin from the avocado and its heart. Chop the avocado instead, season with salt and coriander. Remove lime juice, and stir with a spoon.
13. Bring some of the red pepper mixture onto the plate and top the tuna steaks.
14. Put the avocado salsa on the steaks and garnish with the rest of the red pepper blend.

BOILED QUINOA, CHICKPEAS, AND MOZZARELLA PEPPERS

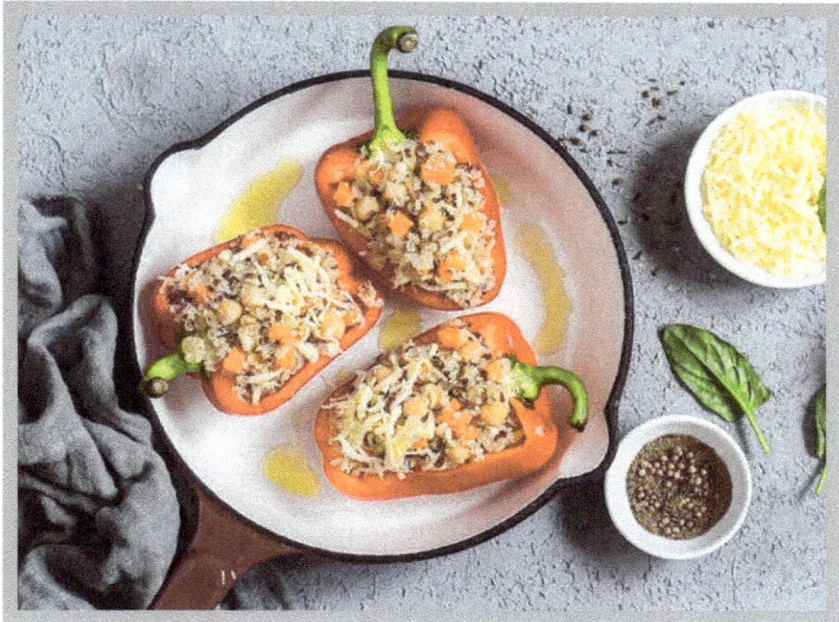

40 MINUTES

Serving 2

KITCHEN-EQUIPMENT
1 workboard,1 knife, 1 saucepan,1 kitchen scale,1 saucepan,1 kitchen strainer,1 saucepan, 1 spatula (wood),1 mortar,1 table spoon.

INGREDIENTS
2 New red bell peppers

QUINOA: 60 g

Shallot 1

100 G / n Carrot

200 g Potatoes

1 Raw Lime

100 G GRATED MOZZARELLA

. . .

1 Cumin Tsp.

1 Black pepper Price

1/2 tsp of salt (salt fleur)

1 1 cup of olive oil

PREPARATION

Put the quinoa in a sieve and rinse with water, then position in a casserole and simmer with water for 6-8 minutes until cooking is finished. Halve the paprika and cut out the heart. Peel the carrot and have it cut into cubes.

Place the chickpeas in a sieve, rinse and drain well. • Cut and dice the shallot, finely. In a bowl of mixtures of olive oil, cumin, pepper and butter, potatoes, chickpeas, shallots and quinoa. Bake the sticky pepper halves for 15-20 minutes in a preheated oven at 175 ° C.

Until eating, drizzle some freshly squeezed lime juice over the boiled pepper halves.

VITAL DUCK, BROCCOLI AND GRANATE SALAD

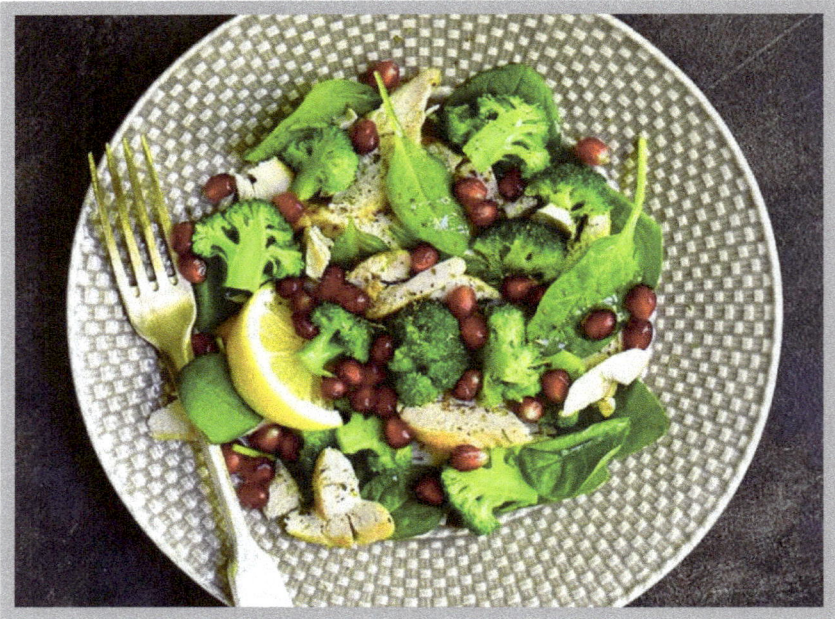

20 MINUTES
  Serving 1

KITCHEN-EQUIPMENT
  1 panel,1 knife,1 panel,1 spatula,1 kitchen scale,1 lemon squeezer
  1 drain strainer, 1 teaspoon.

INGREDIENTS
  120 g breast chicken

BRACCOLI 60 G

60 g Crude Spinach

20 g Grenade

1 TSP of freshly chopped lemon

1 TABLESPOON of salt from the sea (fleur de sel)

1 PINCH hot chili pepper

. . .

Olive oil 1 Tsp.

PREPARATION

Wash the chicken breast with salt and pepper, pat dry and season with butter. • Remove the seeds of the pomegranate from the bowl and set aside.

Wash the spinach, and rinse. Heat the oil in a saucepan and fry the chicken breasts on each side for 4-5 minutes until fried. • Remove the chicken breast from the saucepan and keep warm.

Place preferably on a board, and cover with a second one. • In a hot pan, put the broccoli and fry for 3-5 minutes.

Place the seeds in a bowl of spinach , broccoli and pomegranate and season with lemon, salt and pepper. • Spread it onto a platter. • Cut the breast into thin strips of chicken and scatter over the vegetables.

COLORFUL SALAD WITH CHICKPEAS AND GRILLED PUMPKIN

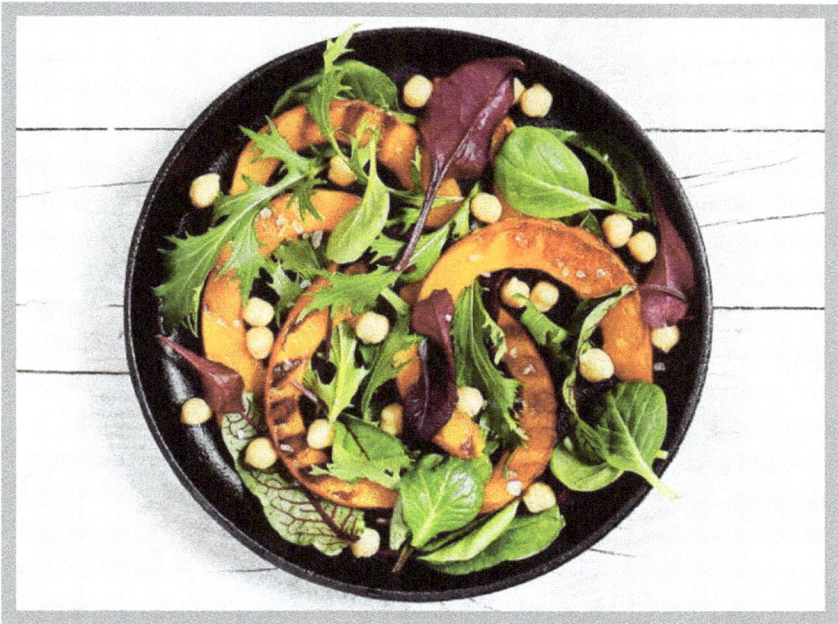

15 MINUTES

Serving 1

KITCHEN-EQUIPMENT

1 Working plate, 1 knife, 1 drainer,1 kitchen scale, 1 grill pan,1 bbq, 1 table spinner,1 salad spinner

INGREDIENTS

100 g Hokkaido casserole

10 g New Arugula

10 GHARD CHARD

10 G ROUGH Spinach

DRAIN 30 G canned potatoes

1 TABLESPOON of salt from the sea (fleur de sel)

1 PINCH hot chili pepper
    1 1 cup of olive oil

· · ·

PREPARATION

Rinse the pumpkin Hokkaido properly, then cut it in half and remove the seeds. • Cut the pumpkin into thin slices, around 100 g. Rinse with arugula, chard and spinach and dry with a spinner on salad. • Put the chickpeas in a sieve and rinse well. Place the lettuce over a pan, and place the slices of fried pumpkin over it.

RED ASPARAGUS WITH AN AVOCADO AND CHICKEN BREAST

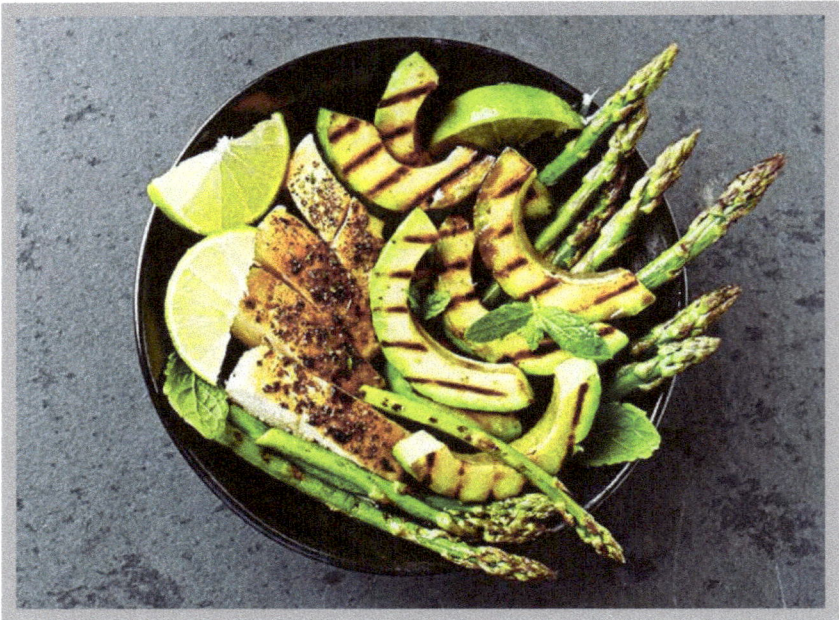

30 MINUTES

Serving 2

KITCHEN-EQUIPMENT

1 work plate,1 knife,1 pot,1 kitchen scale,1 grill pan,1 grill handle,1 lemon squeezer,1 brush,1 table pick

INGREDIENTS

300 g breast chicken

1 NEW HATE at avocado

SPARAGUS: 400 g, black, fresh

1 BRAND freshly squeezed lime

1 PINCH hot chili pepper

1 TABLESPOON of salt from the sea (fleur de sel)

1 TSP, dried thyme

1 1 CUP of olive oil

1 cup of soy sauce

PREPARATION

Rinse breast with chicken and pat dry. • In a container, mix olive oil, soy sauce, lime juice, thyme, sea salt and chili pepper. • Marinate with the meat and allow to soak for 15 minutes.

CLEAN THE ASPARAGUS, and if necessary peel the bottom portion. • Cut the avocado in half and cut heart. • Cut the halves of avocado into slices and cut the peel.

WARM THE GRILL pan and cook the breast on the chicken. • After 5 minutes switching on the water. Now bring the stalks of asparagus and the slices of avocado into the pan.

GRILL IT TILL you remember the roasted strips (then transform asparagus and avocado), and cook the meat through. • Split the chicken breast into strips and combine with sticks of avocado and asparagus.

VITAL SALAD WITH FRIED TUNA, AVOCADO, SPINACH AND GOJI

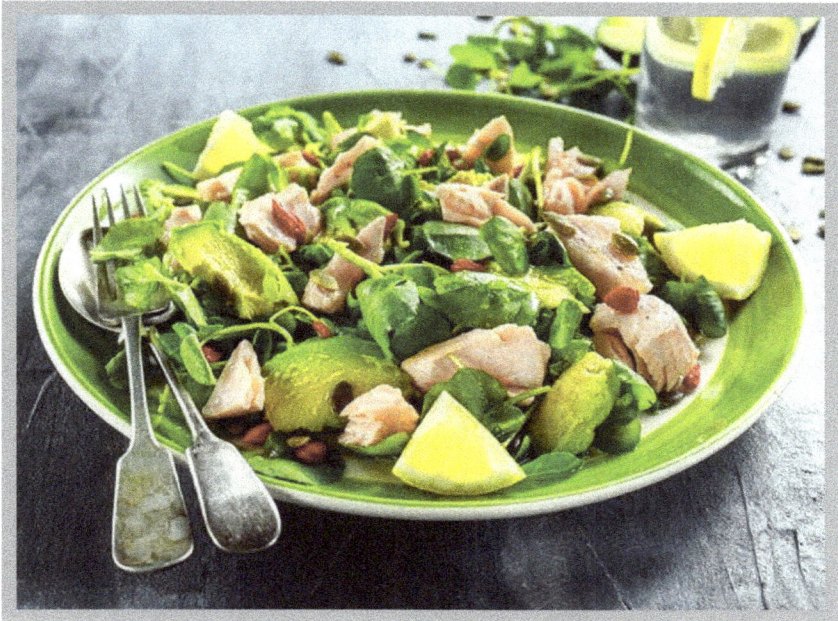

10 MINUTES

Serving 1

KITCHEN-EQUIPMENT
1 chest of drawers,1 knife,1 salad spinner,1 bowl (stainless steel), 1 lemon squeezer, 1 kitchen scale, 1 table spoon.

MATERIALS
50 grams of organic spinach leaves

10 G SALAD with fresh lamb

THREE NEW BASIL stalks

1/2 CLEAN OUTRAGE at avocado

OF COURSE 80 g of tuna fillets in bins

1 Tbsp goji porridge

1 PINCH of sunflower seeds

1/2 Citrus

. . .

1 TABLESPOON of salt from the sea (fleur de sel)
   1 Pinch hot chili pepper

1 TBSP OIL for avocado

PREPARATION

Wash the salad with the spinach and lamb, and dry with a salad spinner, then place on a tray. • Halve the avocado, take half of it out of the bowl, cut into slices and spread over the salad. • Remove from the stalk the basil leaves, and spread the salad over them.

DRAIN THE TUNA, and expanded the salad over it. • Soak the goji berries in a glass of water for a moment, until they are tender. • Spread the salad with the sunflower seeds and goji berries; • Add the avocado oil, lemon juice , salt and pepper to taste, then season.

VITAL SALAD WITH YOGHURT, FLAX AND VEGETABLES

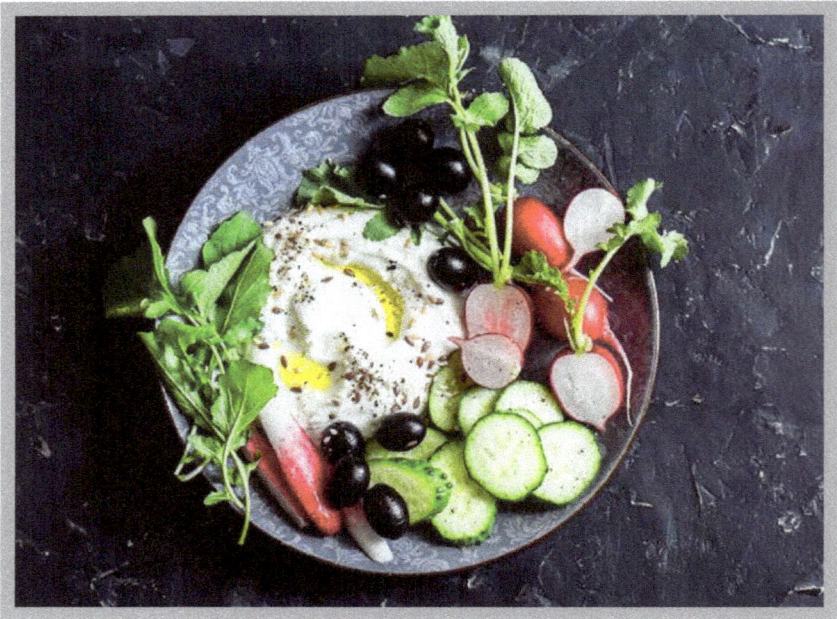

10 MINUTES

Serving 2

KITCHEN EQUIPMENT

1 Working plate, 1 knife, 1 kitchen scale, 1 press of garlic, 1 teaspoon.

INGREDIENTS

e150 g Greek-style yogurt

100 g Cuckoo

100 G CRUDE Radishes

50 GRAMS of Black Olives

1 A GARLIC clove

OLIVE OIL 1 TSP.

1 TBSP. of flax seeds

1 TSP SESAME Light

· · ·

Water salt (salt fleur)

Green Potatoes

PREPARATION
Put the yogurt in a bowl and add in garlic (press the garlic and press the garlic) and olive oil. • Season with salt and pepper to yoghurt.

WASH AND HALVE THE RADISHES • Chop the cucumber into thin slices • Remove the yogurt and serve with the flaxseed, sesame, cucumber, radish and olives.

12

COLORFUL TOMATO SALAD WITH BASIL, MELON AND FETA

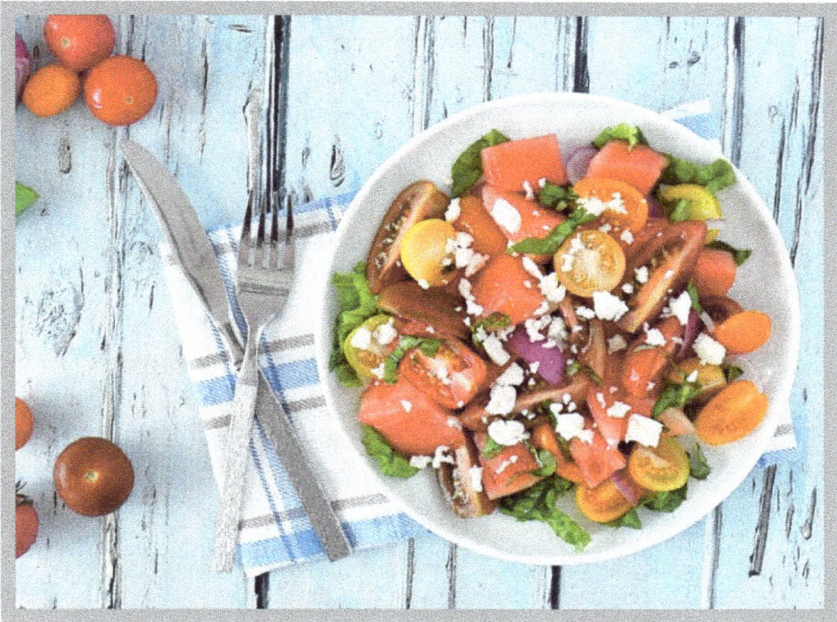

10 MINUTES

Serving 2

KITCHEN-EQUIPMENT

1 Working plate, 1 knife, 1 kitchen scale, 1 lemon squeezer, 1 cubicle.

INGREDIENTS

Cherry tomatoes: 400 g

200 G AQUA Melon

50 G FA.

1/2 RED OINTMENT

5 NEW STALKS, basil

1 RAW LIME, freshly pressed

1 TABLESPOON of salt from the sea (fleur de sel)
2 Spoonfuls of olive oil

.   .   .

PREPARATION

• Cut the melon from the skin and cut it into small pieces • Peel the onion and cut it into thin slices in half • Rinse the basil and pick the leaves from the stalk • Crumble the feta by the hand.

PLACE IT ALL IN A CONTAINER, blend with olive oil and lime juice, and season with salt. • Put in two plates, then serve.

13

GREEN, BACON COVERED ASPARAGUS

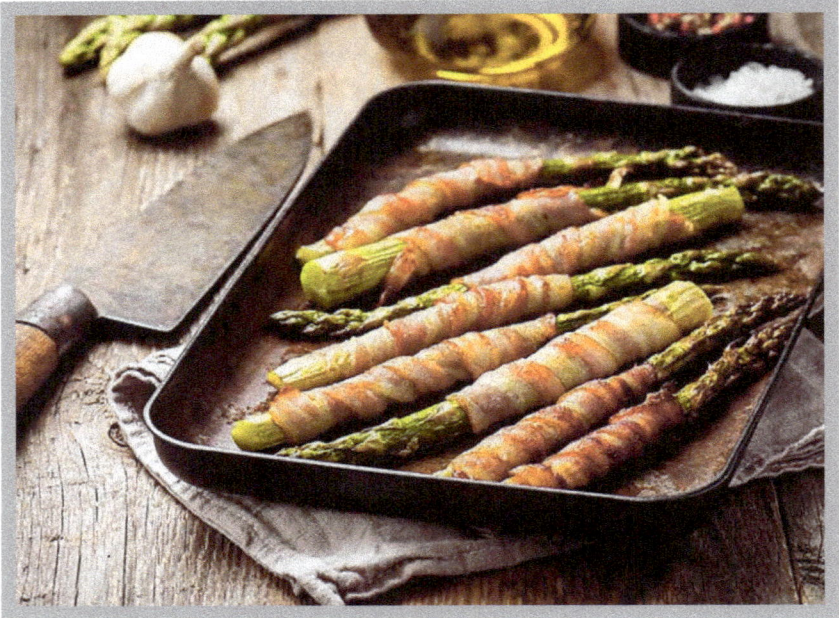

15 MINUTES
  Serving 2

KITCHEN-EQUIPMENT
  1 Tablet, 1 knife, 1 platter, 1 kitchen scale, 1 teaspoon.

INGREDIENTS
  400 g asparagus, green, 200 g fresh bacon with 1 garlic clove

  1 TABLESPOON of salt from the sea (fleur de sel)

  1 PINCH hot chili pepper

  OLIVE OIL 1 TSP.

PREPARATION
  Wash asparagus • Cut the lower third and cut off the ends, depending on the freshness and form of asparagus spears. • Then wrap bacon in asparagus stalks.

  MASH THE GARLIC with the knife's flat side, and combine in a pan and fry with the oil. • Put the asparagus and bacon sticks in the saucepan and fry over medium heat until golden brown.

· · ·

Season with a little salt and pepper to taste. • Remove the asparagus spears from the saucepan and place them on a kitchen towel to absorb the excess fat. Then they serve.

PARMESAN FRIED BROCCOLI, AND ALMONDS

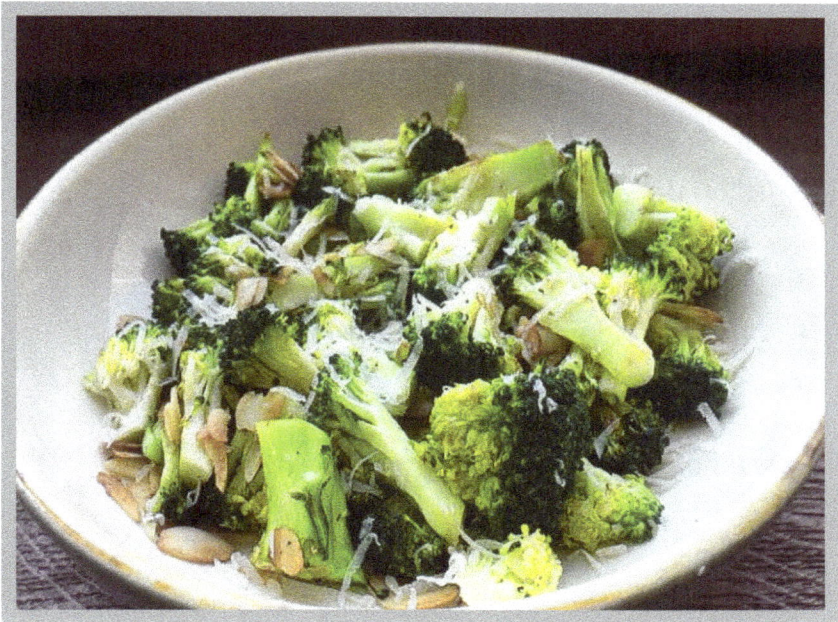

Serving 2

KITCHEN-EQUIPMENT

1 Work plate, 1 knife, 1 casserole, 1 spatula (wood), 1 grater (bowl), 1 cubicle.

INGREDIENTS

500 Grams of Broccoli

30 G ALMONDS with flakes

PARMESAN: 60 g

1 1 CUP of olive oil

1 TABLESPOON of salt from the sea (fleur de sel)

1 PINCH hot chili pepper

PREPARATION

Wash broccoli, chopped off the florets and, depending on their size, halve or quarter them. • The stem can be peeled, sliced into thin slices and put to use. • Parmesan rind.

. . .

ROAST the almond leaves in a saucepan until they are golden brown (without adding oil), then put on a plate and set aside.

POUR THE OIL into the saucepan and cook the broccoli before they bite. • Add the toast almond leaves and thoroughly swirl over them. • Spread the parmesan on two plates and pour over still warm broccoli.

15

HUMMUS CHICKPEA

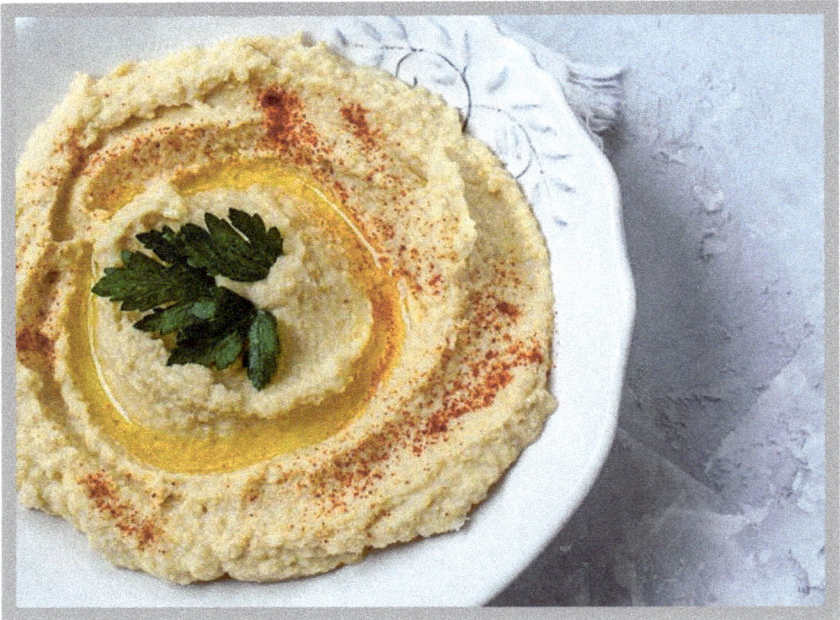

IO MINUTES

Serving 2

KITCHEN-EQUIPMENT

1 workstation, 1 drainer, 1 hand mixer, 1 lemon squeezer, 1 kitchen scale, 1 teaspoon, 1 table cubicle.

INGREDIENTS

220 G canned potatoes

2 TSP, organic tahini sesame

1 A GARLIC clove

5 LBS. of olive oil

TAP WATER ACCORDING to need

1/2 FRESHLY SQUEEZED LEMON / S

2 STICKS of petrol
1 Tablespoon of salt from the sea (fleur de sel)

. . .

1 PINCH hot chili pepper

1 TEASPOON hot powdered paprika

PREPARING

Wash the chickpeas and let them drain in a colander.

BLEND together with a spoon in the freshly squeezed lemon juice and 2 tablespoons of olive oil, and season with salt and pepper.

PUT the hummus on a platter and scatter the remaining olive oil over it. • Brush with the paprika, whisk in the parsley and serve.

16

HEALTHY LIFESTYLE SALAD WITH SQUASH, AVOCADO AND POMEGRANATE DRESSING

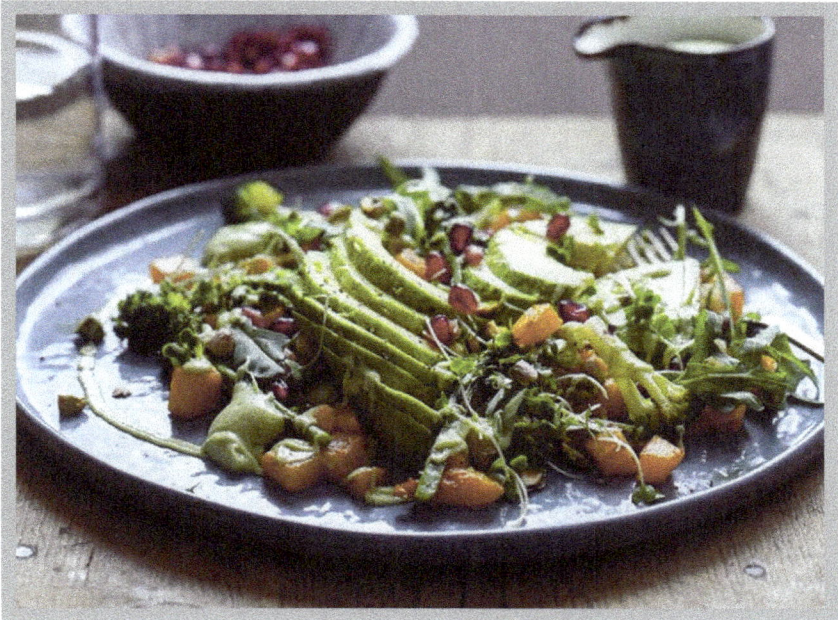

30 MINUTES

Serving 2

KITCHEN-EQUIPMENT

1 panel, 1 knife, 1 casserole, 1 spatula (wood), 1 bowl (stainless steel), 1 sieve, 1 lemon squeezer,1 Kitchen-scale, 1 cubicle, 1 cubicle.

INGREDIENTS

1 New hate at avocado

30 g Grenade

Hokkaido pumpkin 60 g

BRACCOLI 60 G

20 G RABBIT

2 TSP BRAND new cress

3 Split almonds

. . .

40 G YOGURT, 1.8 per cent of course

1 TSP SWEETHEART
   1 Brand freshly squeezed lime

1 TBSP OIL for avocado

1 TABLESPOON of salt from the sea (fleur de sel)

1 PINCH hot chili pepper

PREPARING

   Cut the avocado and take the core off. • Strip the skin pulp, and cut it into slices. • Cut the lime and suck the juice out. • Drizzle the lime juice to the avocado pulp.

RINSE THE PUMPKIN and dry it, then cut in half and remove the seeds with a spoon. • The pumpkin is processable without peeling. • The pumpkin is sliced into small pieces.

WASH BROCCOLI, cress and arugula, and drain. • Slice the broccoli off the stem. • Heat the oil in the saucepan and fry the knob. • Remove broccoli, and quickly fry.

• • •

ADD SOME AVOCADO, lime juice, salt , pepper and honey to a beaker and puree using the hand blender for the dressing yogurt.

PLACE ONTO A PLATE THE AVOCADO, arugula, pumpkin and broccoli. • Add the chopped almonds, cress leaves and pomegranate seeds and add a little salt and pepper to season. • Dress and serve

17

EGGS SCRAMBLED IN LOW-CARB BREAD

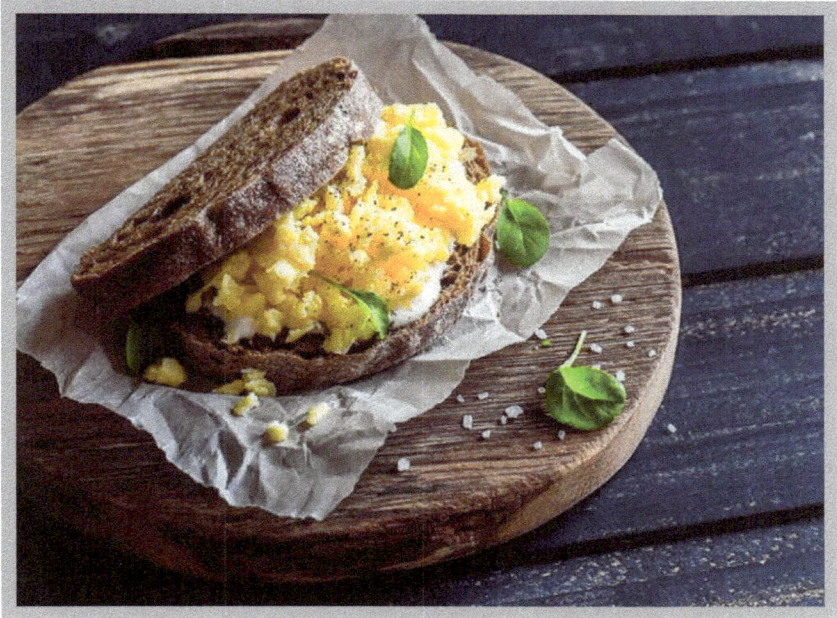

10 MINUTES

Serving 2

KITCHEN-EQUIPMENT
1 wall, 1 knife, 1 bowl (stainless steel), 1 whisk, 1 grater, 1 skillet, 1 spatula (wood), 1 teaspoon.

INGREDIENTS
2 Cheese bread slices

SIZE M. 2 EGGS.

20 G GRANULAR CHEESE

10 G PARMESAN cheese

OLIVE OIL 1 TSP.

1 TABLESPOON of salt from the sea (fleur de sel)

1 PINCH hot chili pepper

1 FRESH BASIL Stem

· · ·

PREPARING

In a container, grate the parmesan and whisk the whites, then season with salt and pepper. • Heat the oil in the saucepan, add the eggs and let chill on moderate heat. • Use the spatula to work through the egg mixture, so that it is prepared evenly.

Layer the bread with the granular cream cheese and layer the scrambled eggs over the end. • rinse and dry the basil, pluck the leaves and garnish the scrambled eggs.

18

VITAL BOWL OF QUINOA, AVOCADO, SPINACH, CHIA AND ALMOND SEEDS

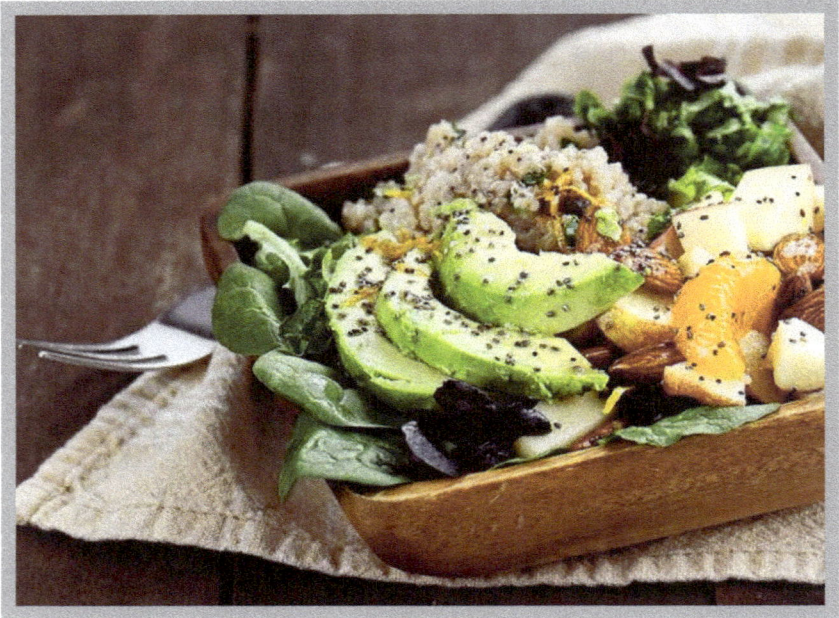

20 MINUTES
Serving 2

KITCHEN-EQUIPMENT

1 knife, 1 pot, 1 wooden spoon, 1 lemon squeezer, 1 kitchen scale, 1 cup, 1 salad spinner, 1 mortar, 1 table spoon.

INGREDIENTS

Fifty g quinoa

1 NEW HATE at avocado

40 G LEAVES of organic spinach

30 G ROMANESQUE salad

20 G RABBIT

Apple 1

1/2 HALF ORANGE

. . .

10 Mandarins

1 Tsp seed chia

2 Tsp raw sprouts

Olive oil 1 Tsp.
   ½ Lime, newly squeezed
   1 Tablespoon of salt from the sea (fleur de sel)

Preparing

Wash the quinoa cleanly under cold water in a colander and cook for 8-10 minutes in a small pot filled with water. • If the quinoa is still somewhat firm, drain the water and allow the granules to evaporate into the pot. • Then a quinoa with some freshly squeezed lime juice water and a slice of salt to taste.

Wash the leaves with lettuce and dry them in a spinner for salad. • Split the avocado in half, remove the peel and cut the pulp into thin slices. • Rinse the apple or peel it, and cut it into small bits.

Use the orange to cut off the extract and filet the pieces with the knife. • Place the sprouts in a sieve and rinse away. Then let it drain on them. • Put the bits of almond, orange and apple together in a container.

DIVIDE THE SALAD into two saucepans. • Spread the fruit salad and quinoa over the top. Simply add lime juice and olive oil to the avocado and drizzle over. • Apply the chia seeds as a finishing touch.

19

NICE BOWL FULL OF QUINOA, AVOCADO, BROCCOLI AND SPROUTS

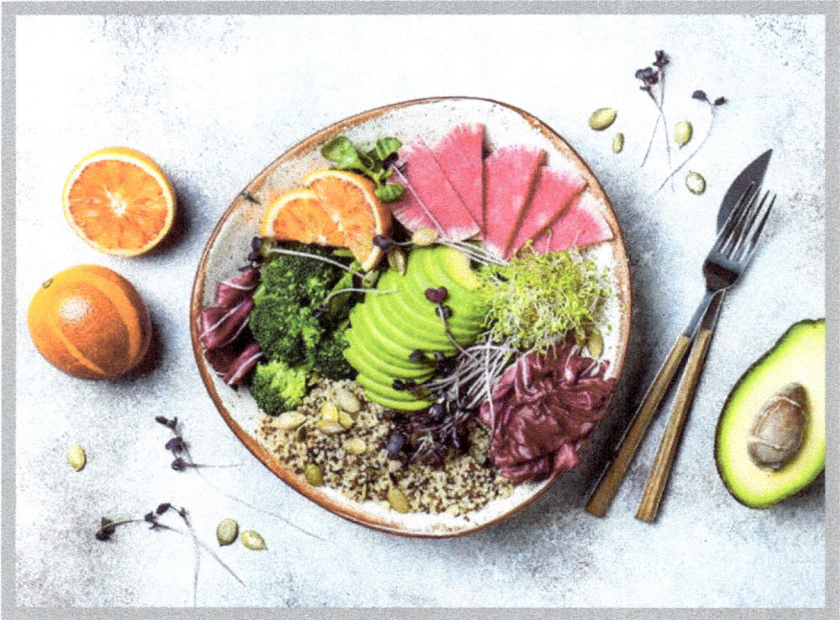

20 MINUTES
Serving 2

KITCHEN-EQUIPMENT

1 kitchen strainer, 1 knife, 1 pot, 1 wooden spoon, 1 lemon squeezer, 1 kitchen scale, 1 table spoon.

INGREDIENTS

50 g, raw quinoa

1/2 LAWYER

BROCCOLI 100 G

60 g Crude Beetroot

1/2 HALF ORANGE

RADICCHIO 30 g.

IT SPROUTS 5 g of alfalfa

. . .

ROUGH 5 G of radish sprouts
   1 Brand freshly squeezed lime

2 TBSP PUMPKIN SEEDS, incomparable

2 SPOONFULS of olive oil

1 TABLESPOON of salt from the sea (fleur de sel)

1 PINCH hot chili pepper

PREPARING

Wash the quinoa cleanly under cold water in a colander and cook for 8-10 minutes in a small pot filled with water. • If the quinoa is still somewhat firm, drain the water and allow the granules to evaporate into the pot. • Then a quinoa with some freshly squeezed lime juice water and a slice of salt to taste.

TRY TO WASH THE BROCCOLI, briefly separate the small flowers from the stem and steam. • Cut and halve the beetroot and cut into thin slices. • Halve the avocado, remove the pulp from the bowl and cut into thin slices with a spoonful.

·   ·   ·

SLICE THE ORANGE, then cut it again in half. • Rinse the radicchio and cut into pieces between 2-3 small leaves. •Wash the sprouts under runny water in a fine strainer.

PLACE it all in two bowls, put olive oil and pumpkin seeds and add salt and pepper to the seasoning.

20

CAULIFLOWER BAKED WITH WALNUT PESTO

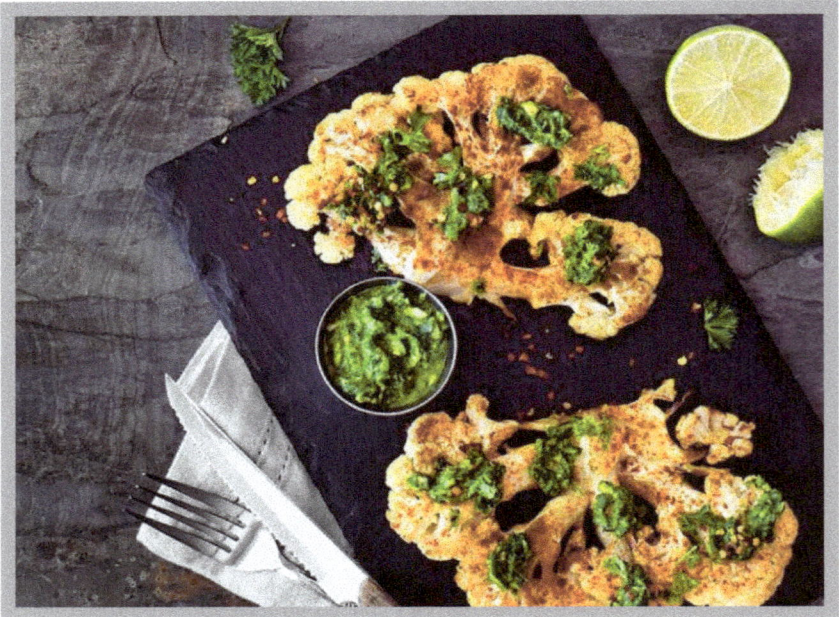

40 MINUTES

Serving 2

KITCHEN-EQUIPMENT
1 Working plate, 1 knife, 1 hand blender, 1 kitchen scale, 1 lemon squeezer, 1 baking paper, 1 cubicle, 1 teaspoon.

INGREDIENTS
1 kilogram cauliflower
80 g Kernel walnut, new

6 PETERSIL STALKS

6 FRESH STALKS, basil

OLIVE OIL: 100 ml

40 G PARMESAN cheese

1 A GARLIC clove

1 BRAND freshly squeezed lime

. . .

1 Tsp of salt (salt fleur)

1 Pinch black chili pepper

Pimentón de la Vera: 0.5 g

1 Tsp flakes of chilli

Preparing

In a convection oven preheat the oven to 160 ° C. Rinse and cut the cauliflower into approx. Slices 2 cm thick. In a cup, place 2 spoonfuls of olive oil, Pimentón de la Vera, chilli flakes, salt and pepper and blend. Place a baking sheet covered with baking paper (two baking sheets may be required) and bake for approx. 25-30 minutes.

Wash the basil and parsley and shake dry, put all herbs in a blender jar (with stems). • Extract the garlic, and attach the walnut kernels in the bottle to the herbs. Stir the remaining olive oil in slowly. • Blend parmesan now and add to pesto. Then, mix again briefly. • Season salt, pepper and lime juice to the pesto. Put the cauliflower baked on the plates and serve with pesto.

21

PANGASIUS IN ASIAN THEME

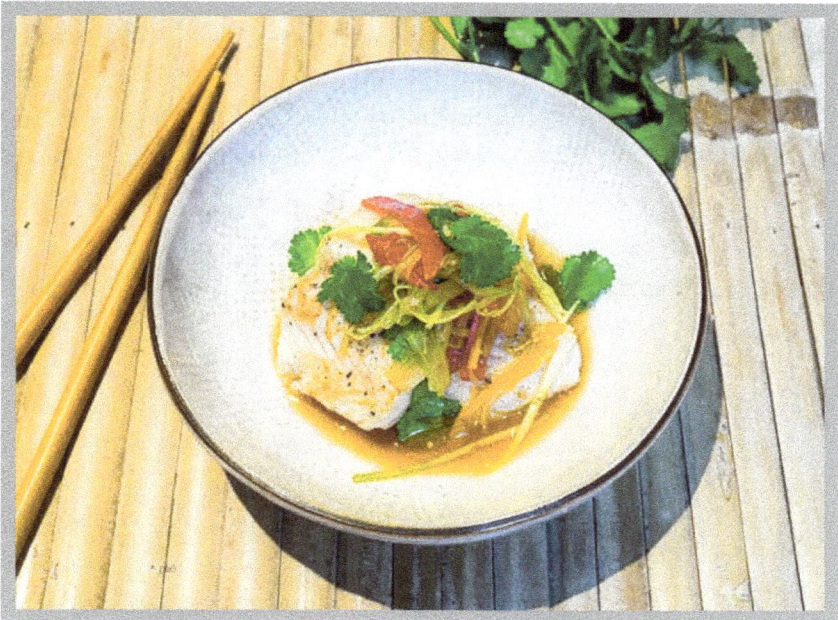

15 MINUTES

Serving 2

KITCHEN-EQUIPMENT
1 Knife, 1 work board, 1 pan, 1 cubicle.

INGREDIENTS
120 g Crude pangasius

1 TBSP OIL for avocado

100 G CRUDE chili peppers

40 G (RAW CELERY), raw celery

10 GRAMS of spring onions

40 G ROUGH Leek

6 CILANTRO STALKS, new

1 Pepper ginger

. . .

2 CUPS of soy sauce

20 ML NEW orange juice

2 TSP SIRUP agave
    2 Pinch salt

½ Crude Lime

PREPARING

Rinse the vegetables, and drain. Discard from the peppers seeds and partitions, and cut them into very narrow strips. • Cut the stick of the celery into very short strips. • Clean and cut the spring onions into very tight strips.

SPLIT THE PORK into rings that are very close. • Squeeze half of the lime out and mix the juice in a bowl with soy sauce, orange and agave syrup. • Finely rub the ginger over the grater. • Season with salt and add bell pepper, celery and spring onions.

CHOP THE PANGASIUS fillet into pieces. • temperature the avocado oil in a pan and fry the pangasius across both sides for almost four minutes. • Clean and shake dry cilantro, then pluck the seeds. • Add the fish and pour the cilantro leaves over the salad.

22

BAKED SWEET POTATO SALAD WITH AVOCADO AND KALE

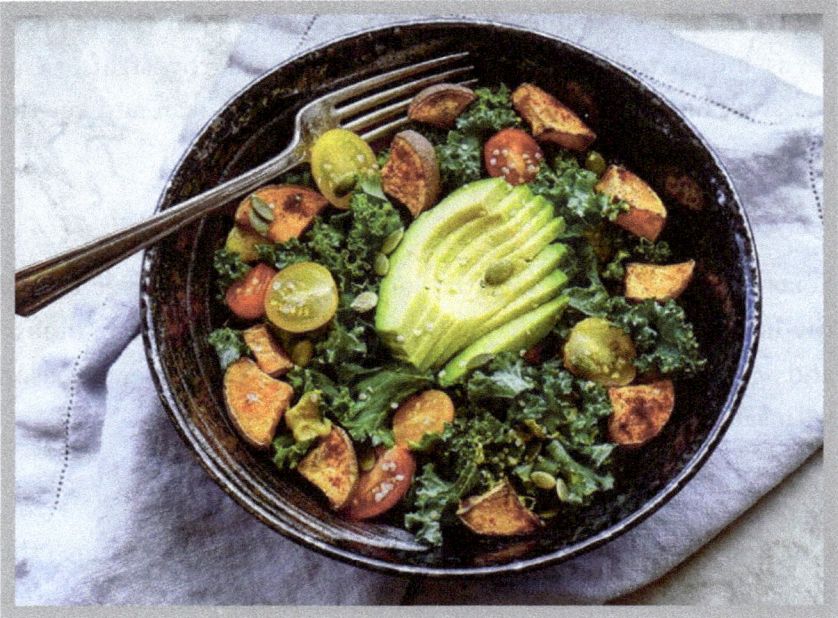

Serving 2

KITCHEN-EQUIPMENT
1 Work plate, 1 knife, 1 salad bowl.

INGREDIENTS
Kale: 150 g, fresh

100 g Sweet Kitten

100 G CHERISHED tomatoes

100 G of new hatred at avocado

2 MEZZANINES of olive oil

1 PINCH of salt from the sea (salt fleur)

1 PINCH black chili pepper

1 PINCH of Pulverized Paprika

. . .

1 PINCH of Powdered Turmeric

PREPARING

Delicious   sweet potatoes can be eaten in a container. •
rinse and dry the sweet potatoes . If you doesnt like it with a
mug, remove them. extract   the sweet potatoes into pieces and
put them on a baking sheet lined with baking paper • Bake the
potatoes 10 to 15 minutes in the preheated oven.

WASH THE KALE, and drain it well. • Wash the tomatoes, and
halve them. • Cut the avocado in half, remove the core and cut
the pulp into slices. • Put the tomatoes and kale in a salad bowl.

STIR in the olive oil and add the paprika and turmeric powder,
salt and pepper. • In bowl, add the oil mixture to the kale and
mix together. • Add slices of avocado and finally add the warm
sweet pieces of potato in the oven.

BREADED CHICKEN BREAST WITH QUINOA AND GRILLED VEGETABLES

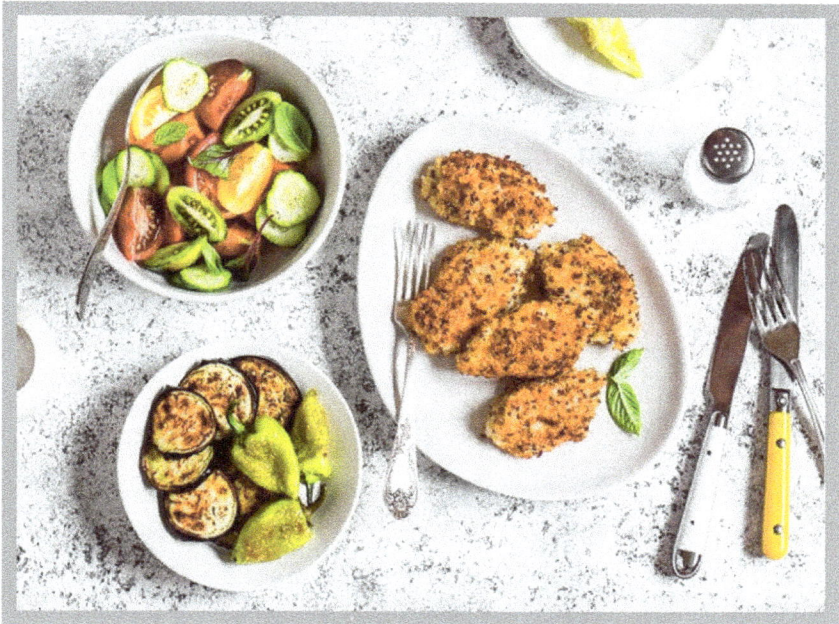

40 MINUTES
  Serving 2

KITCHEN-EQUIPMENT

1 work desk, 1 knife, 1 pan, 1 grill tongs (stainless steel), 1 kitchen scale, 1 baking dish, 1 bowl (stainless steel), 1 table cubicle.

INGREDIENTS

300 g breast chicken

50 G COOKED Quinoa

1 SCALE of an egg M.

150 g Crude Aubergines

200 G NEW PINK, small bell peppers

TOMATOES: 200 g / s

Curdy 200 g

. . .

1 PINCH of salt from the sea (fleur de sel)

1 PINCH hot chili pepper

1 SLICE of Pulverized Paprika

2 SPOONFULS of olive oil

Preparing

Wash the breast of the chicken, pat dry, cut into small pieces and fry with salt and pepper. • In a bowl , beat the egg and whisk with a fork; • Add salt and pepper and stir in the chicken. • If the meat is well absorbed by the liquid egg, add the quinoa and fry pieces of meat with it.

PREHEAT THE OVEN with circulating air up to 100 ° C. • Heat the oil in a saucepan and fry the meat for 2-3 minutes, until golden brown on each side. • Place the meat in a baking dish and cook over the middle shelf in the oven.

WASH THE EGGPLANT, season with salt and paprika, cut into slices, then return to the pan (where the meat was fried) and slightly brown. • wash and fry the pepper with an eggplant; Then turn off the oven.

. . .

WASH TOMATOES AND CUCUMBERS • Cut the cucumber into slices and quarter tomatoes • Put them all in a bowl, season with salt and pepper and a little oil.

REMOVE the meat from the oven and serve with the vegetables as well as the tomato and cucumber salad.

24

KITTEN POUND WITH SAGE BUTTER

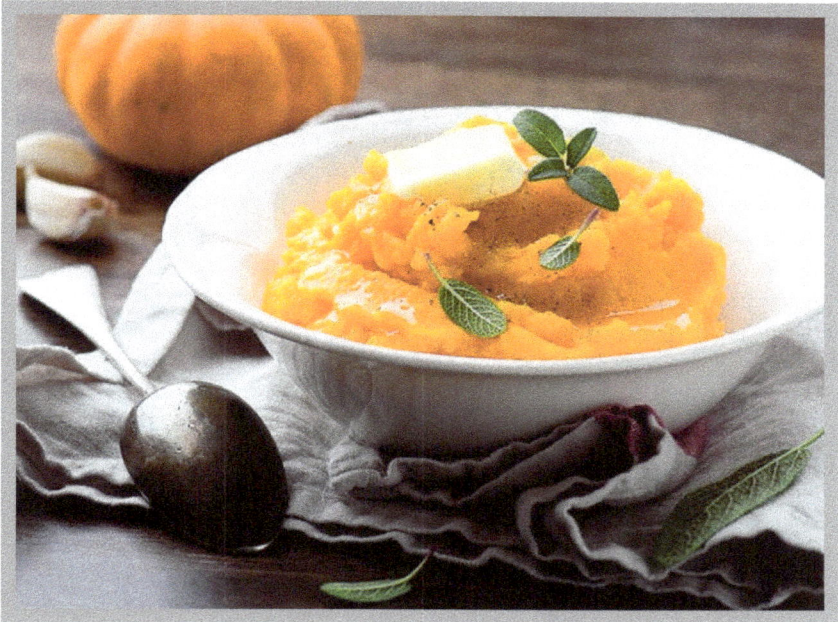

40 MINUTES

Serving 2

KITCHEN-EQUIPMENT

1 Working board, 1 knife, 1 pot, 1 wooden spoon, 1 kitchen scale, 1 potato masher, 1 bowl, 1 cupboard, 1 teaspoon.

INGREDIENTS

Hokkaido 500 g Pumpkin

BUTTER: 60 g

2 FRESH-SAGE STALKS

2 GARLIC NAILS

1 PINCH of dried mustard

ONE TSP of turmeric powder

1 TSP of salt (salt fleur)

1 PINCH hot chili pepper

Preparing

Cut the Hokkaido pumpkin open and remove the seeds and fibres. • It is advisable to remove the peel with mash or puree, as it is too difficult to hammer and rather uncomfortable to notice. • Slice the pumpkin into cubes of about 2 cm after peeling.

IN A SAUCEPAN , bring the water to a boil, add a little salt, stir and then add the cubes of pumpkin to the saucepan. • Simmer the pumpkin for 15-20 minutes, until it crumbles soft but not.

Increase the temperature of the butter in a small saucepan and allow it to dissolve, afterward add the garlic (melt down the toes with the knife's flat side) but also add the sage leaves and fry them over moderate heat. • Check that the butter does not burn or turn black.

PRESENTLY DRAIN out the pumpkin water. Simply add the sage butter to the pumpkin and mash it with a potato masher until you achieve the desired consistency. • Add the turmeric, salt and pepper, then season with nutmeg.

SALAD WITH PROTEIN FLAKES, ROASTED

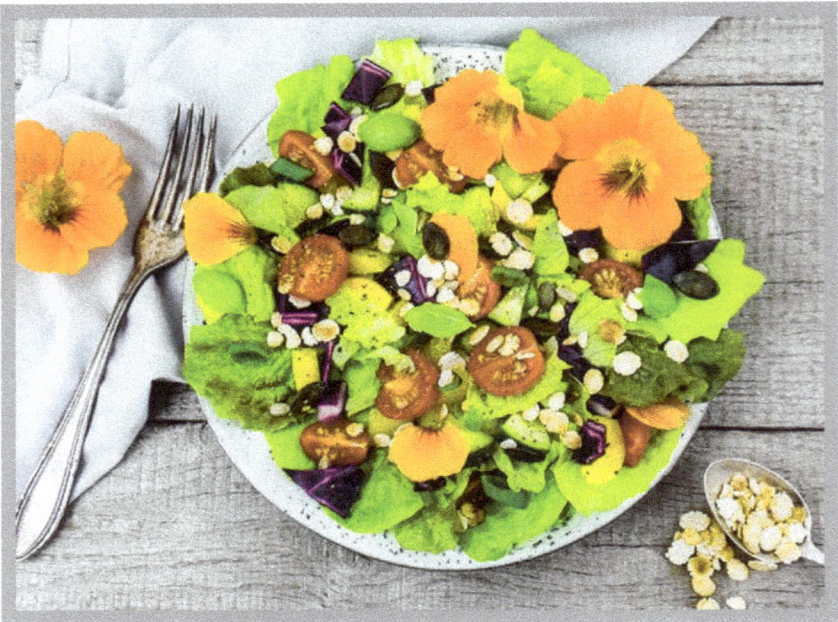

10 MINUTES

Serving 2

KITCHEN-EQUIPMENT
1 Knife, 1 Tablet, 1 Panel.

INGREDIENTS
50 g Lettuce roman

Five Cherry Tomatoes

25 G YELLOW POTATOES

25 G ROUGH Red Cow

50 G CURTAINS

1 1 CUP of olive oil

15 G of soca protein flakes (de-oiled soya flakes)

15 G KITTEN seeds

. . .

1 NEW BASIL Stem

1 PINCH MARINE salt

1 TABLESPOON hot chili pepper

PREPARING

Fry the protein flakes from Socas in a saucepan without adding fat. • Wash the leaves of lettuce and allow to drain well. • Then pluck the leaves of lettuce into pieces and put them on a platter.

RINSE THE TOMATOES and the rest of the vegetables and rinse. • rinse the basil, and dry it. Then pluck your leaves. • Have the tomatoes halved. • sliced the cucumber into pieces, bell pepper and red cabbage.

APPLY THE SALAD WITH TOMATOES , cucumbers, chili peppers and red cabbage. • Season with olive oil to the salad. Simply add Socas protein flakes, pumpkin seeds (or other seeds as you like) and basil leaves to the salad and add salt and pepper to season.

HINT: Edible flowers such as the nasturtium give a visual focus.

26

FOOD PREP-LOW CARB COURGETTE PASTA WITH PARMESAN SHRIMP SAUCE

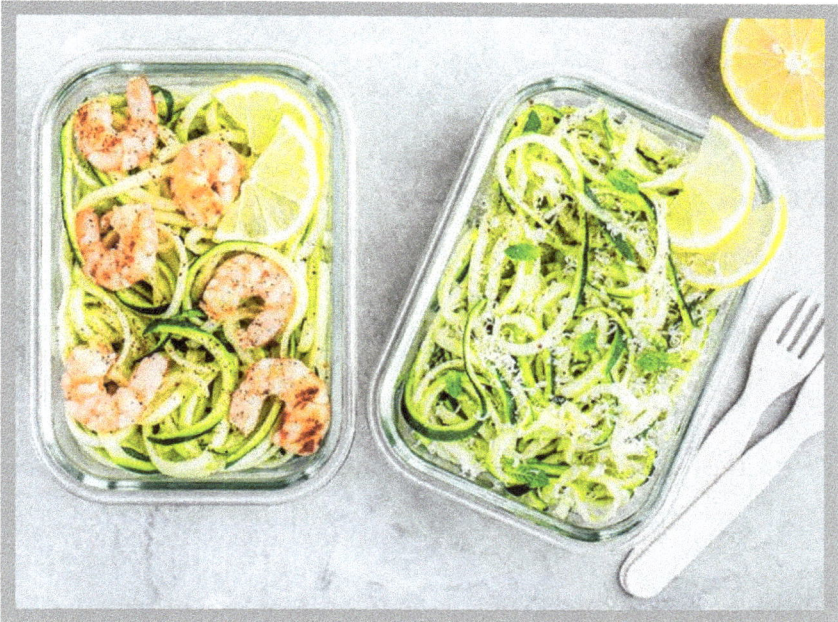

20 MINUTES

Serving 2

KITCHEN-EQUIPMENT

1 knife, 1 spiral cutter, 1 kitchen scale, 1 garlic press, 1 bowl, 1 wooden spoon, 1 teaspoon.

INGREDIENTS

400 g courgettes

200 g Skinless Garnelas

PARMESAN: 60 g

½ Citrus

1 A GARLIC clove

1 PINCH of salt from the sea (fleur de sel)

1 PINCH black chili pepper

1 CUP BUTTER

4 Seasoned olive oil

PREPARING

Scrape the garlic and press it into a medium sized bowl using the garlic press. • Add olive oil, lemon juice , salt and pepper and stir in a fork.

CLEAN THE ZUCCHINI, dry them out and slice it into long , thin pasta using the spiral cutter. • Heat the saucepan with a bit of oil, add the prawns and fry them on the both sides till golden brown.

TAKE the prawns out of the saucepan and add a little bit of butter and oil. Simply add half of the rubbed parmesan and allow to simmer shortly, after this stir in the zucchini.Poured the zucchini pasta in two cans or jars, using the shrimp. • put extra can of the remaining parmesan. • Heat the whole in a casserole, sprinkle the parmesan over it and serve.

27

CHICKEN SPROUTS WITH NEW HERBS

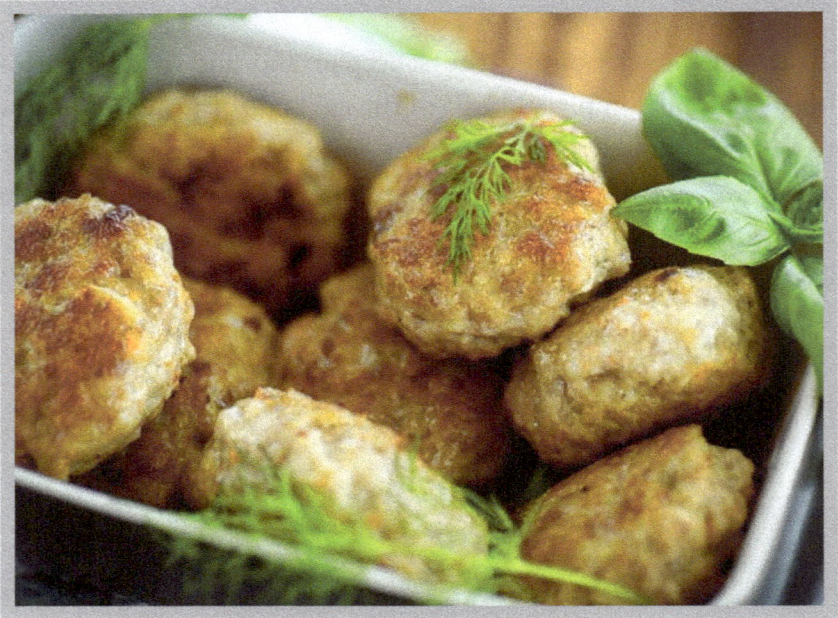

30 MINUTES
Serving 2

KITCHEN-EQUIPMENT

1 working plate, 1 knife, 1 casserole, 1 spatula (wood), 1 bowl (stainless steel), 1 garlic press, 1 kitchen scale, 1 teaspoon.

MATERIAL

500 g breast chicken

1 TABLE LITRE of yogurt in Greek style

2 TSP MEDIUM mild mustard

2 SHOALS

1 A GARLIC clove

1 EGG YOLK, chicken egg Size M

4 NEW STALKS, basil

· · ·

2 FRESH DILL Sticks

1/2 TABLESPOON CUMIN

1 TSP of salt (salt fleur)

1/2 TSP BLACK chilli
   11 cup of olive oil

PREPARING

Spin the chicken breast or finely chop it with a knife through the meat grinder. • In a bowl, put the chopped chicken, add the yogurt, egg yolk, mustard and the spices.

SCRAPE THE SHALLOTS, dice them thinly and fry them in a little oil, again add them to the minced meat. Simply remove the garlic, then press the garlic and add to the chopped meat. • clean the basil and dill, shake dry and chop thinly, then add to the hazelnuts.

KNEAD all by hand with a fork, or the latest. • cleanse your face, slightly moisten and then form tiny meatballs from the mixture. Heat the remaining oil in the saucepan. • Fry both sides of the meatballs till golden brown, and serve.

· · ·

THESE MEATBALLS often taste very nice cold, and can be well cooked as a meal.

28

LOW CARB SPAGHETTI WITH TOMATO AND LENTIL SAUCE

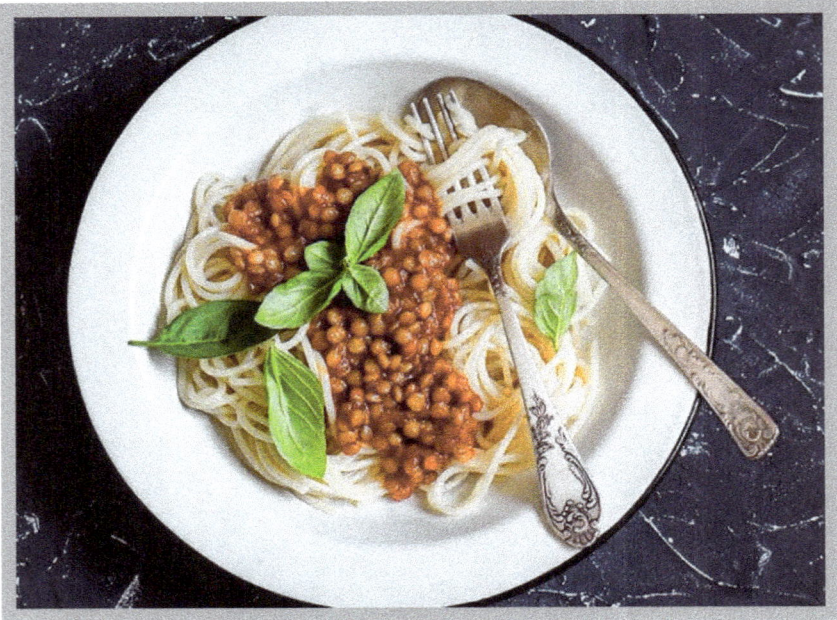

30 MINUTES

Serving 2

KITCHEN-EQUIPMENT

1 knife, 1 kitchen scale, 1 kettle, 1 wooden spoon, 1 kitchen strainer, 1 lemon squeezer, 1 table spoon.

INGREDIENTS

100 g Spaghetti with low carbide

40 g Lentils

Shallot 1

1 A GARLIC clove

PASSATA 200 ml

FRESHLY SQUEEZED 1⁄2 Lemon

2 STALKS of fresh basil

200 ML VEGETABLE BROTH, homemade

· · ·

2 TBSP BALSAMIC vinegar (Aceto Balsamico)

I TABLESPOON of olive oil

I PINCH of salt (fleur de sel) 1 pinch of salt

Preparing

Heat the broth, and let the lentils cook for 10 minutes. • realistically, drain and use the broth in a cup for other purposes. • Stir the lentils under the balasamic and lemon juice, and season with salt and pepper.

SCRAPE AND CHOP the shallot and garlic, and fry. • Add passata, and briefly bring to a boil. • Put the lentils in the sauce and add a bit of broth if appropriate. • Sprinkle with salt and pepper.

HEAT up the pasta in salted water, as instructed in the box. • Drain and put on plates. Simply add the pasta lentil sauce and garnish with basil, then serve.

29

CHICKEN BREAST WITH SAUCEPAN

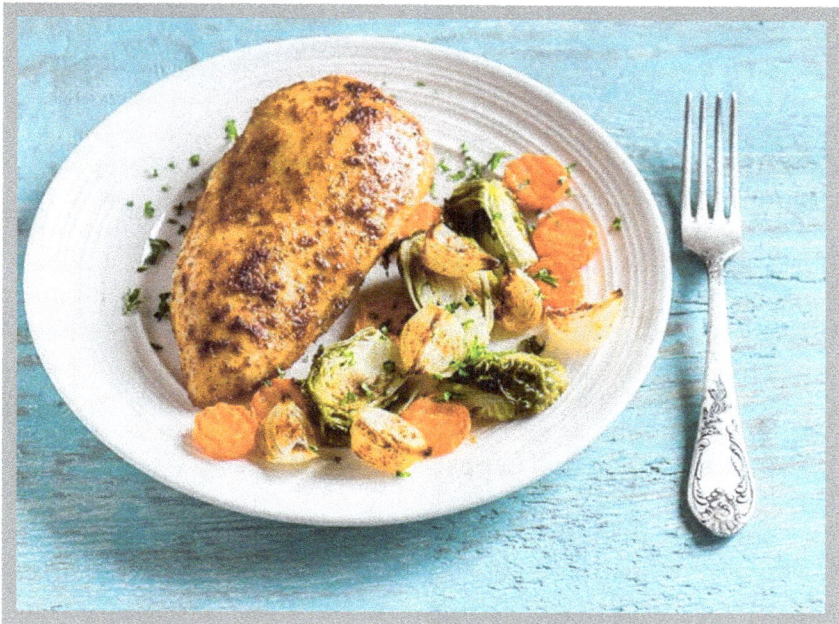

30 MINUTES

Serving 2

KITCHEN-EQUIPMENT

1 Working plate, 1 knife, 1 pan, 1 grill lock, 1 kitchen scale, 1 table-litter.

INGREDIENTS

180 g skinless breast chicken

EIGHTY G of Brussels sprouts

120 G / n Carrot

120 G / n Onion

1 TABLESPOON of salt from the sea (fleur de sel)

1 TABLESPOON hot chili pepper

1 1 CUP of olive oil

1 PARSLEY STEM, fresh

. . .

PREPARING

Wash and pat dry chicken breasts • Remove the dry stem and withered leaves from the Brussels sprouts and cut them in half.

SCRAPE AND SLICE CARROT • Peel onion and cut into bits • Clean parsley and shake warm, then chop.

HEAT the olive oil in the pan and fry the chicken breasts till golden brown on both sides until the meat is cooked. • Season with salt and pepper over the chicken breast.

PLACE THE VEGETABLES in the frying pan, then season with salt and pepper. • Can the chicken breast on a plate with the potted vegetables and sprinkle with the parsley.

www.ingramcontent.com/pod-product-compliance
Lightning Source LLC
Chambersburg PA
CBHW071116030426

42336CB00013BA/2103